Her Hair Is Her Crown of Glory!
Lessons and Strategies for Growing Your Beauty Shop

Alan D. Benson, MBA, MPA

I Dare You to Do It Right Series

Benson Group, LLC
c/o MHB Publishing
101 North 7th Street
Louisville, KY 40202
Alandbenson.com

Table of Contents

Dedication

I dedicate this book to all of the women in my life.
You exemplify the highest example of womanhood,
and for that, I respect and honor you.

Your Hair is Your Crown of Glory!

**I Corinthians 11:15: "But if a woman has long hair,
it is a glory to her: for her hair is given her for a
covering."**

Preface

Hello, and thanks for picking up this book, Her Hair Is Her Crown of Glory! Lesson and Strategies for Growing Your Beauty Shop. I am also the author of Keep that Seat Hot! Strategies of Operating and Growing your Barbershop. I am excited about both books because they are about the stylist becoming a better operator, manager and leader both in business and the community. I am a businessman and educator who has taught barbers and beauty shop owners about managing and marketing a business; and because of that, I have helped many of them improve their operations. I credit this skill to my academic background, management experience, and overall, the gift God has given me. Aligning those three qualities has been a journey for me. It took self-reflection of who I am, experiencing failures, conducting an inventory of my gifts and determining what drives me. From my reflection, I came to the calling that I need to help people improve their lives through their businesses. So, this book is all about helping you to achieve your business goals.

What inspired me to write this book on the beauty shop? I know that a woman's hair is not just a part of her physically, it is also attached to her emotionally and mentally. Equally important, the beauty shop is a part of my life experience. I experienced it as a son to my mother, brother to my three sisters, and father to my daughter. The beauty shop has been and still is a stable business in our society and is a $43 billion industry. Being a stylist is a respectable profession where primarily women come together to cut, reshape, extend or color their crowns. I have looked at beauty shops through the lenses of both the customer and the business owner as salon owners have taken my business courses. I have seen the good, bad and ugly as they relate to the industry. I have talked with several salon owners about their marketing, financial futures and business acumen throughout the years. For those reasons, I was inspired to write this quick and easy, how-to book. This book is a manual that equips stylists and beauty shop owners with the tools to operate, enhance and grow their business.

You will find this book to be straight-forward, easy-to-understand, and clear in its instructions and examples. The title indicates that a woman's hair is her crown of glory, and that she seeks to treat it as such. In order for her to keep her hair as a crown, she needs to go to a beauty shop that will provide her the royal treatment.

Acknowledgements

First, I would like to thank God for giving me the insight, spirit and drive to write this book. My personal experiences, both positive and painful, have helped to shape who I am today. Thank you, God! Second, I uplift my mother, Marthella H. Benson, who inspired me beyond belief. I remember my first experience being inside a beauty shop was with her. Our church member, Ms. Streeter, was her stylist, and to keep me still, Mom would always buy me a 7-Up to drink. I would be so happy to get that 7-Up and to spend alone time with my mother. Those were the days. Mom is no longer here, but her spirit and teachings live within me. She always pushed me to be a better man and to hold myself accountable; she always dared me to do right. For that, the books that I write are part of the I Dare You to Do It Right! Series.

I also would like to thank my father, Sam D. Benson.
He is my hero because he is a man of faith, strength and achievement. I thank my sisters, Janet, Pam and Stephanie. Growing up with you showed me the qualities that women of class, grace and eloquence

should possess. I am thankful that you all are still around, and I love the family gatherings and great cooking that we share. I would like to thank Bryan of Elegant Image and Lissa of All Phases Salon for sharing their perspectives on working in the beauty shop industry. I thank my friend, Kevin Haggard, Sr. – MBA, CFP, for sharing his perspective on creating financial stability for barbers and stylists. Kevin and I met when I was president of the National Black (MBA) Association, Inc. – Kentucky Chapter, and I appreciate his insight and wisdom. Thanks, Rhonda, of Perk It Up Salon for keeping it real with me; I appreciate your insight and judgement. I want to thank my barber, Donte, the owner of Beyond the Cuts Beauty Shop in Louisville, KY, for his continuous support. Donte and I grew up on the same street and I am thankful for his friendship. To this day, we laugh about the things we used to do. I am really proud of Donte's deliberate pursuit in achieving his vision to grow his business and make the community a better place. Finally, I would like to thank Yvonne R. Jackson, my editor. Here we go again! I appreciate your professionalism and attention to detail.

Introduction

Natural hair, short hair, extended hair, relaxed hair: all these conditions show a woman's versatility. Black hair, brown hair, blonde hair, red hair: all these colors express how she feels. Natural flat twists, crochet braids, rod sets, high buns, Marley twists, faux locs: they all show the differences in her life. The people who style hair are both women and men. Most enter the profession immediately after high school, and some come back to their passion of styling hair after completing college and having successful careers in other areas. Former counselors, accountants and business majors decide to enter into this industry. Why is this so? They are passionate about the business, and beauty shops are an integral part of the booming beauty industry! Internationally, the beauty industry is a $425 billion industry. In the United States alone, it is a $43.7 billion industry. To paint a picture of how behemoth the beauty industry is in the U.S., it is over 11 times larger than the U.S. barbershop industry, which has sales of $3.7 billion.

To account for the $43.7 billion, haircutting and styling

are over 57 percent and coloring 23 percent of the business. The other 20 percent accounts for resale of merchandise, cosmetics, skin-care products or services, and other related services.

My first introduction to beauty shops occurred when I was a child. I would go to the beauty shop with Mom. Going to this shop was quite different from going to the barbershop with Dad because the women did not have much to say. On the other hand, my father and his friends would talk about everything, and I am sure it was filtered. Nonetheless, the conversations were limited because I was in their presence. Like the barbershop, the beauty shop was filled with various magazines and books I always enjoyed reading, such as Ebony and Jet Magazine. Those fondly remembered experiences have passed, but the congregation and socialization at the beauty shop are still present.

The beauty shop is an important fixture to communities, and some would argue that it is recession-proof because both men and women need and like getting their hair cut and styled. Because of the need, the value it can bring customers, and its historical foundation, the beauty shop presents many business opportunities if strategically planned and executed. The business opportunity that a beauty shop can offer involves owning and operating a business, selling products in the shop and creating personal wealth. It is hard work, but like anything, if you put your time into it, it can be rewarding. Owning a beauty shop presents many benefits. You will have the autonomy and freedom of ownership and the opportunity to create wealth, but most importantly, you help women restore, reshape and create their crown.

The goal of my writing this book is for you to be more knowledgeable and equipped to own and operate a lucrative beauty shop business. At the end of each chapter, I have questions for you to answer to help you self-reflect about your business. These questions will help you organize your thoughts and execute your plan. Owning and operating a business requires some skill, discipline and know-how, but can be accomplished. To alleviate a few headaches, this book will take you through the necessary steps in operating and growing your beauty shop.

Even while corporations are taking away some of the beauty shop business and individuals are facing barriers of entry into the hair care supply chain, I will explain why the beauty shop business is still a growth business and what one needs to do to ensure that his or her business sustains itself. For example, having the shop at the right location to create and sustain business growth is essential.

The next chapter goes over steps on how to become licensed and how to run an operationally efficient and effective beauty shop business. I have heard many stylists say, "This is my part-time gig!" Your beauty shop might be a part-time gig, but you could be missing out on a huge opportunity in creating a business empire. Think about what you are doing, put the pieces together, and focus on making your beauty shop reach its full potential. This is such a great opportunity! I remember attending a conference where a bank executive stated, if he were not in banking, he would be in the beauty shop business. Why did he say that? Because he recognized the financial opportunity and stability the beauty shop industry presents.

I will then discuss operating your beauty shop business and having the right people on your team. Having the right people on your team can grow your business just as well as having the wrong people can kill it. As the owner, you are the leader of a team and it is up to you to set the tone and direction of your business. In any business, you must have the right support; therefore, I will give tips on hiring practices. the right team members for your business is critical to your success. I also will discuss things to avoid such as money mismanagement. Money mismanagement will break the backbone of any business. Your money management style will dictate whether or not your business is going to remain open, expand, invest or close. I will give strategies for maximizing your revenue and ways to control cost. I also will discuss strategies on pricing. Using your money to prepare for your future will also be discussed. I will discuss paying self-employment and payroll taxes, disability insurance, business insurance and life insurance. Your money, if used wisely, will propel your beauty shop to new heights.

The "If I Build It, They Will Come" section will cover strategies for marketing your beauty shop. This is an important section because it will give you tips and suggestions on how to market the products and services in your beauty shop. This section will cover the 4 Ps of marketing: product, price, place and promotion. I also will discuss the branding of your beauty shop. Branding is a special logo, a slogan, a name, a product look or a way of providing service that people will identify with your beauty shop. Branding is very important because it differentiates your beauty shop from others. For example, when people see the golden arches, they immediately think about McDonald's.

Being your customer's keeper is another important aspect of running a business. In this section, I will discuss customer service and what it means to provide excellent customer service. The reality is that without customers you will not have any business. In addition, providing bad customer service is a recipe for killing your business. I guarantee that! I will discuss strategies for getting, keeping and growing your customer base. Customer service is so important to the growth of your beauty shop that regardless if you had a bad day or restless night, when your beauty shop opens, it is show time and you have to put your game face on.

We all look at reality TV and sitcoms and see the huge

homes, fancy jewelry and beautiful cars. The "Real Housewives of Atlanta," "Empire," and even the "Wheel of Fortune" would have us believe that everyone leads a glamorous life. The media present glitz and glamour that appeals to us all. In this section, I will discuss how having the right curb appeal will attract more customers. This is a section that turns into marketing, branding and overall strategy in maintaining and growing your beauty shop.

Using the right technology and planning are critical steps in owning, operating and growing your beauty shop business. The following chapters tell what technology is available to assist your business in becoming more operationally efficient and what steps to take to turn your beauty shop into a corporation of beauty shops throughout the city, state, or nation. Enjoy this reading!

Chapter 1
Why Is The Beauty Shop a
Growth and Stable Business?

The beauty shop and its services have been a part of our history. It can be traced back to 4000 BC when historians found that Egyptians used beauty products such as kohl to create dramatic eyes. In the 19th and 20th centuries, women revolutionized the beauty industry. One such person, Elizabeth Arden, built a cosmetic empire. By 1929, she owned 150 upscale salons across the U.S. and Europe. Her 1,000 products were found in the luxury markets in 22 countries. She was the sole owner, and at the peak of her career, one of the wealthiest women in the world (Wikipedia, 2017). During that time, the need for products and services for African-American women became in more demand. Annie Malone founded and developed a large empire that centered on cosmetics for African-American women. While she was coming of age, the popular style among Black women was that of a "straight hair" look. Black women were starting to turn their backs on the braided cornrow styles associated with the fields of slavery and began to embrace a look which, for them, meant freedom and progression toward equality

in America. By the beginning of the 1900s, Ms. Malone began to revolutionize hair-care methods for all African Americans. Armed with a revolutionary formula and a product she called "The Great Wonderful Hair Grower," Ms. Malone moved to St. Louis in 1902. She hired some assistants and began selling her products door-to-door. Word of her products and teaching method spread like wild fire and soon her products and her "Poro Method" of styling hair were a success. Malone believed that if African-American women improved their physical appearance, they would gain greater self-respect and achieve success in other areas of their lives. One of Annie Malone's employees was Madame CJ Walker (Annie Turnbo Malone African-American Educator, Entrepreneur & Inventor, 2017).

Annie Malone was recorded as the United States' first black millionaire with assets of $14 million in 1920, and she was the owner of Poro College. Poro is a West-African word meaning "physical and spiritual growth." Poro College was a five-story facility that had a manufacturing plant, a retail store that sold products, a 500 seat auditorium, a roof top garden, and business offices. The college was for black women. She wanted the women to learn the skill of cosmetology as well as give back to their communities. While many people have not heard of her, she is considered the mother of the hair care and cosmetic industry. The college also employed nearly 2,000 people in St. Louis, and through its school and franchise businesses, her business created nearly 75,000 jobs for women in North and South

America, Africa and the Philippines.

Another mother of the hair industry was Madam CJ Walker. Seeking treatment in 1905 for her hair loss, Madam CJ Walker created the "Walker System;" a system used for scalp preparation, application of lotions and ironing combs. She had the gift for self-promotion with a personal touch, which propelled her business to empire status. She employed more than 3,000 workers, mainly salespeople who sold door-to-door to black women (http://www.history.com/topics/black-history/madame-c-j-walker, 1991). As time progressed, the industry steadily grew.

The Numbers

Today, the beauty salon industry alone is a $43.7 billion industry and it is steadily growing. It is expected to grow to $48.5 billion by 2022. In 2017 alone, sales increased by 1.5 percent. Along with providing cutting, styling and coloring, there are other products and services that compliment beauty shops. For example, according to IBISWorld report, organic, natural, and eco-friendly products are expected to become more prominent by 2022. This will create more demand for products and services for eco-friendly products. Women between the ages of 20 and 64 use the beauty shop and its services because of their disposable income. Women between the ages of 35 and 44 account for 27 percent of industry sales. Women, 45 to 55, account for 23 percent. Women between the ages of 25 and 34 account for 16.5 percent, and women between the ages of 55 and 64 account for 15.7 percent of sales. Those over 65 account for 9.7 percent, and those 25 and under, 8.1 percent of sales.

The Market

Entry into the beauty shop industry is not difficult; however, there is a lot a competition. The industry is fragmented and no company dominants the market. According to IDIS World report, the top four companies account for less than 10.0% of industry revenue. The largest company in the industry, Regis Corporation, generates just 3.3% of total revenue and is still 60% larger than the next-biggest company.

Within the industry, hair stylists give haircuts, style hair, apply hair coloring and provide scalp treatments. Hairstylists are also trained to perform manicures, pedicures and eyebrow shaping. Hairstylists advise clients about hair care techniques and help to sell salon products to clients. Hair stylists can enjoy careers in the entertainment industry at salons, spas and cosmetology schools, or as freelance stylists. Most states require stylists to be licensed. Licensing could involve a one-time exam or application in some states, while others require continuing education credits or periodic re-certification. They usually need a high school diploma or GED to apply to cosmetology school and typically graduate in nine months to a year with an associate degree in cosmetology. In some states, cosmetology programs are offered in high school. It is recession-proof because, despite the economy, women will find the resources to get their hair cut and styled.

Employment and Demands of Beauty Shop Stylists

Entering the beauty industry presents many opportunities for growth and wealth. Overall employment and demand for stylists was projected to grow 10 percent from 2016 to 2026. This is faster than the average rate of growth for all other occupations. This demand is directly connected to the population growth and the need for hair-care services. In addition, depending on the demographics of the population, the demand could be greater.

Basically, this percentage increase indicates that there is a need for this occupation and needs spell opportunity. To capitalize on this opportunity, one must have a plan, be at the right place and location and acquire the resources to make it happen. So, how do you start with a plan? It's simple because we all are equipped with an imagination. Whatever you imagine for your business, write it down on paper and type or speak it into your smart-phone. This plan will be a very rough draft, and you will add to it, remix it, and take away from it before you have a final plan. One important step is to put your plan in a business plan. A business plan maps out how you're going to operate your business. If you need to finance your business, you must have a business plan. There are various organizations that can help you with your plan. You need to seek out some level of assistance or wise counsel to determine if you can put your plan into action. If you already know how to put your plan in place, you have accomplished a great task. I will caution you about sharing your ideas with others. Share your ideas with only a few trusted people in your circle. After you have a solid plan, determine what resources you will need as well as the cost for you to start your beauty shop. An important part of getting your plan in place is looking for the location for your beauty shop. The location is important for driving business and customers to your beauty shop; this will be discussed in a later chapter.

Shifting Attitudes

According to IBISWorld Industry Report 2017 for Hair Salons, "Over the past five years, salons began to cater to specific demographics. Male hair care is one of the fastest-growing haircare segments, thanks to trending hairstyles, such as the fade, which requires upkeep and more frequent visits to the barber. Overall, there has been a paradigm shift in male attitudes toward grooming and self-care over the five years to 2017. This change was primarily reflected by increased male grooming product sales."

A Stylist's Income and the X factor

According to the Bureau of Labor Statistics, a stylist's median income (in the middle of pay range) is $12.38 per hour. The lowest 10 percent earned less than $8.62 per hour, and the highest 10 percent earned more than $23.58 per hour. Depending on the vision of the stylist, many stylists earn much more than the national averages. While those figures give you medium salaries, I believe that the amount you earn is dependent on many factors. I call it the X factor. Your market (city), target customer, strategy, brand and vision all are factors. However, the X factor is when stylists make the decision to take their business to greater heights and they are driven to achieve it. The X factor is something that you can't teach. You can have all the education and latest styling products or the biggest salon, but your success is determined by what is within you. I have interviewed and talked with several barbers and stylists, and they are doing quite well. Some are making thousands of dollars per week, but don't be fooled; they are putting their time in it, have mastered their craft and are disciplined. They are at their place of business early, often leave late and have a consistent book of clients. They take their business seriously! This way of doing business parallels all businesses and successful people, in that they have a method and discipline to achieving their goals. Don't get it mistaken that they don't have drawbacks; however, they use their drawbacks as tools to keep pushing forward.

Questions

- Why are you in the beauty shop business and what do you expect to get from it?
- What are your financial goals?
- Where do you see yourself and your business in 10 years?

Chapter 2
Transforming Your Beauty Shop from a Hustle to a Legitimate Business

Styling hair is something that many of us have the capability of doing, and some of us have styled hair in the past. Being the youngest of three sisters and one brother, I have witnessed my mother doing my sisters' hair. Growing up, my sisters did not have the luxury of going to a salon until they were teenagers. Having three daughters going to the beauty shop would be costly, so our mother would press their hair with a pressing comb. Mom was very careful during this process because with one wrong move one would either mean burnt hair or a screaming child. As you could imagine, it was an all-day process, and while it may have saved money, I believe she would have gladly paid someone a few dollars to help save her the time and energy involved in an entire day dedicated to hair. This is just one example of how people become connected to the industry by styling their hair or younger siblings' hair to help save money and realize that they have a talent. It is the perception in both the barbering and beauty shop communities that doing hair is a great side hustle, something to make some extra money. This is puzzling because being a stylist in a beauty shop is an excellent profession to expand and grow a business. It is a great opportunity. I have talked to salon owners throughout the U.S. that have fabulous places of business. They are clean, comfortable and well run. I see the stylists as not only operating within their craft, but having a creative side because of all the different types of styles that they provide. It is all in how you view it. Many opportunities are in front of our faces and while our eyes are physically open, we must determine if something is an opportunity for us or not. You can dig into it by determining the pros and cons and whether your skill set aligns with the opportunity. What plagues us sometimes is that we have so much going on that we want immediate gratification and to make as much money as soon as possible. The reasons for that vary. It could be because of family obligations or the need and quest to be rich, but whatever the case may be, I do believe that we should take a step back and look at where we are, what we're doing, where we're going, and where we need to go.

The first step in transforming your hustle into a

legitimate business is becoming a licensed stylist and an owner and registering your business with federal, state and local governments. Your registration at the state level is setting a business structure. There are many forms of business structures, but the most common forms of beauty shop business structures are Sole Proprietorship, General Partnership, Corporations and Limited Liability Company (LLC).

Sole Proprietorship

A sole proprietorship is a business that is owned by a single individual. It is the easiest type of business structure to form because no paperwork is needed to file with the state unless you want to run your business under a name different from your own. A license or permit and registration of business with your local government might be needed. This is attractive to many because their businesses will not be bogged down with government regulations; they also do not have to deal with oversight of partners, boards or shareholders. Sole proprietors also can report their income on their personal taxes.

A major disadvantage of a sole proprietorship is that as

the business owner, you are personally liable for any debts that the business incurs, and   if sued, you are personally liable. That means all your assets (home, car, etc.). In addition, it can be very difficult to get a bank loan as a sole proprietor.

Depending on your type of business, I would be a little hesitant to operate as a sole proprietor, primarily because of the liability. I was at a conference and this millionaire businessman said that once you start making money, you will become a target for others. People will come after you and your assets. I believed him. Take precautions to protect your personal assets.

General Partnership

A general partnership is the same thing as a sole proprietorship.   The difference is that a sole proprietorship involves only one person; a general partnership involves two or more people. Therefore, a little more work must be done to divide the business responsibilities and ownership percentages between both owners. Like the sole proprietorship, no paperwork needs to be filed with the state unless you want to operate under a different name.

The key drawback of a partnership is that you are personally liable for any of your partners' mistakes. For example, if one of your partners accidentally injures a customer, both of you will be held liable, which can affect your business and personal assets.

Having a partner can be a win-win situation for you both. I have been in salons and have talked with a number of husbands and wives in business partnerships. Personally, I think that is powerful because there is nothing like a couple building a business together. Even in this case, however, I would advise that each partner's role and every detail of the business be spelled out in a contractual form and to purchase insurance.

Purchasing insurance could save a lot of heart ache and loss to your business. For example, a partner could be killed in an accident, leaving the other partner with uncomfortable business decisions to make. I have worked with people who developed partnerships with their current love interest and/or best friend, and that is a great partnership when business is good. On the other hand, I would add that when businesses are challenged by personal tragedy, declining health, or economic recessions, it is easy for friendships to break down; therefore, having a clear understanding of each other's role in the business and a clear understanding on the direction of the company are critical.

Corporation

A corporation is a business entity that is recognized as a separate legal entity from its owners. A corporation is a complexly different business structure. They are more complicated to set up and understand than sole proprietorships and general partnerships. Corporations have ability to conduct business, sue or be sued. Unlike the previous two business structures, actual paperwork is required. A common form of a corporation is an S Corporation.

An S Corporation, commonly called an S Corp, is a special corporation under the IRS tax election. Under this system, the profits and losses can pass through to your personal tax return and the business is not taxed. Only the owners of the business are taxed. This protects the corporation from double taxation. Corporations are taxed as a separate entity as well. There are tax savings benefits to this structure, but it does make business setup a bit more complicated.

The owners of a corporation are called shareholders. The primary ad- vantage of having a corporation is the limited liability it grants its shareholders. What that means is an owner is only liable up to the amount he/she has invested in the business. Another benefit of a corporation is that it can implement a benefit and profit-sharing program for its employees.

Limited Liability Company (LLC)

The Limited Liability Company (LLC) is a business structure that acts as a corporation but is not one. It is not a corporation, but it can still provide the corporate like protection that is important for many business owners. An LLC can act to be taxed as a sole proprietorship, partnership, or S Corporation, and income and expenses can simply be passed through to the members' (owners) individual tax returns.

In all the cases, it is extremely important to your business to not mix your personal money with business. How you run and operate your beauty shop is another way of how you can transform it from a hustle to a legitimate business. How you treat your customers, your finances, the activity that takes place inside and alongside your business, and even the patrons of your beauty shop will tell the story about your business. It might be a perception to some customers, which could be their reality. The marketing and the finances of your beauty shop will be discussed in a later chapter.

Questions

- If you think your business is a hustle, what will it take for you to change your mindset?
- What is the best business structure for you?
- What perception do you want to give your customers about your business?

Chapter 3
From Legitimacy to Growth: Creating a Business Model

The beauty of owning your own business is that you are in total control of how it looks and where it's going. The pleasure to me in being a business owner is the ability to dream, and to put a vision in place that is going to help people. What I found is that often we come up with our vision from our experiences, both positive and negative, and we turn those experiences into power. When I say power, I'm saying it could be something that could change the face of the community or create a need for a customer base. So, in laying the foundation for your business, you must look at what direction you're headed and forecast where you see it in 5, 10, 15, and 20 years. Some might look at this as a little crazy because we don't know where we're going to be 20 years from now; however, we need to think ahead in everything we do regarding our life and business. For example, you might plan to own 20 different beauty shops regionally 20 years from now. You also might plan to sell your beauty shop to another company in 10 to 15 years. Those are legitimate plans a stylist could put in place, and the sky is the limit with one's planning and investment for their business. So, in making this investment, how do we know if we are making a right business move? Are you selling just because of the dollar amount; or is the dollar amount offered a fair market value for the investment? To safeguard our beauty shop business, we need to develop a business model to ensure that we get a fair Return on Investment (ROI).

A business model is how you're going to operate your beauty shop; the direction it is going; what type of clientele you are to service; what type of services you're going to offer; and the list can go on and on. Your business model is taken from your experiences coupled with your know-how in running and operating a business. While owning and operating a business might be a new venture, I would advise that you seek wise counsel to assist you with developing the appropriate business model for your company. There are many services that can give you advice, both free and paid, regarding what resources are needed, what direction your company should go, and how it should be grown. I would advise that once you get your business filed and make it legitimate, exercise wisdom with whom you do business and from whom you receive wise counsel. When your business is on fire with growth, you're going to have other companies that will solicit your business, claiming to be experts in their field, when in fact, they are just another company looking to make money from you and give you a lot of false hopes and false dreams. Always do your research on a possible service provider as well as check references.

Many might think that a business model is the same as a business plan; however, it is not. A business plan outlines the operations of a company. A business model outlines how and what way your company will function. It plans out its day-to-day operations. A business model describes the company's position within the industry value chain and how it organizes its relations with potential customers. This would position your beauty shop to maximize revenue as well as profit. So, how do you develop a business model for your beauty shop?

For starters, look at what products and services you're going to offer while planning out your beauty shop. I have been in many beauty shops throughout the years. Many offer various styles and cuts, as well as beverages and snacks. That is all fine and dandy; however, there are still other great opportunities out there for a stylist to make money in addition to cutting hair. So when developing your vision for your beauty shop, develop a list of what services and products you would like to offer in addition to cutting hair. For example,, a business model of traditional beauty shop services could include the following:

- **Hair Styles:** Cut and style, relaxers or permanent straightening methods, keratin treatments, one-step hair color, highlights, toner, corrective color, hair and scalp treatments
- **Natural Hair Services:** Offering various styles and conditioning for maintaining and stimulating women's natural hair; one-step hair color, highlights, toner, corrective color
- **Nails:** Manicures, pedicures, paraffin
- **Hair Removal Services:** shaping, waxing, laser treatments
- **Men's Services:** Haircut, beards, and grooming
- **Skincare Services:** Essential facials and peels, sports massage, deep-tissue massage

A non-traditional business model service, would be having a beauty shop and the option of a tax service during tax season. This setup would offer tax services to customers as they wait to get their hair styled. I think this is a great and creative business model. Another business model that could be in a beauty shop is having an expanded retail line of women's clothes as well as products. These clothes could range from dresses, suits, shoes, and much more. When it comes to expanding a product line in a beauty shop, the sky is the limit. I will say that with expanding and having a retail line it is also important that you stay on top of your inventory so that you do not lose items, money, or potential profits. You can attach almost any product or service to the beauty shop as it relates to your customers. You can have a childcare service in place while your clients receive their services. You can provide a meditation and yoga room for your customers. Whatever the case, I would do my research and study what customers need in addition to hair styles. When you do that, you will be able to better determine what products and services you're going to put into your beauty shop.

In conclusion, developing your business model for your beauty shop will require time, effort and money. I would carefully think about what products or services to offer, in addition to just styling hair. The prices of products and services could really be profitable for your beauty shop if purchased at a reasonable price and sold to your customers. Develop a list of products and services you would like to provide, their costs and the prices you're going to charge. This would be a great starting point in planning your business model.

Questions

- How do you see your beauty shop operating?
- How will you determine what products and services fit your customer base?
- What types of customer services would you like to offer?
- What types of customer products would you like to offer?

Chapter 4
Having the Right Team in Your Beauty Shop

In life, we all have been equipped to have great imaginations and ideas. Some of us have the inherent instinct of leadership while others have different abilities. We are equipped with great ideas and visions. As we move our business forward to another level, we must have the right people and teams in place. Having the right people and team in place will propel your business to greater heights, and the wrong people will sink your business into failure. In developing your beauty shop and positioning it to go to a new level, determining the right people and building the right team is paramount. Here's what I mean by having the right team.

Having the right people in place is key to carrying out your expectations for operating an excellent business. Those expectations should include how to provide excellent customer service to all customers.

Another expectation is having a professional look and presentation to your customers, such as all team members wearing solid black with a stylist cape or in uniforms with beauty shop logos. As a form of promotion, your team might sport different hairstyles to show your customers styling options. Your team would also be responsible for maintaining beauty shop rules and etiquette, such as no smoking or profanity while in the business.

You must establish how you want your team members to look and how you want them to treat your customers. With that said, you cannot discriminate against any potential team members; however, if they do not possess that skill set or meet the qualifications, they do not meet the standards of being on your team.

Finding the right people for your team requires an interview process. The interview does not have to be anything formal, but it needs to happen. This interview process should consist of the potential team member completing an application that lists his/her experiences as a stylist, credentials and references. This will help you to determine their qualifications, skills and abilities. During the interview, ask various questions about servicing customers, working on teams, handling different styling situations and handling conflict from dissatisfied customers. Below are sample questions to ask and avoid during an interview.

Questions to Ask

Can you tell me more about yourself as a stylist? What types of customers do you like working with?

Satisfactory Response in telling more about yourself: If the stylists tell you they are just completing school or they have been in the industry for a while.
Unsatisfactory Response: The stylist tells you, "I don't really know what to say about me or there is not that much to say about me."

Satisfactory Response with working with customers: "I enjoy working with all customers. I have worked with all ages; and I style for women and cut men's hair."

Unsatisfactory Response: There is not an unsatisfactory answer because a stylist might only work with a certain client base and earn a certain amount of money. For example, "My clients are executive women."

What motivated you to become a stylist?

Satisfactory Response: This answer could vary because everyone has different motivations for why they choose this field. Even if a person says to make a lot of money, that is an acceptable answer.

Unsatisfactory Response: There is really not any unsatisfactory answer because it is the interviewee's opinion.

What are your goals in becoming a stylist?

Satisfactory Response: While this is an opinion-based question, people's goals differ. What you want to look for in this question is if the interviewee's goals align with your goals.

Unsatisfactory Response: Not having any goals is not a good thing; however, this is not a deal breaker. The person could be young and need some guidance and mentorship. I would weigh this response with how the interviewee answered all the other questions.

What is your ideal type of customer and beauty shop?

Satisfactory Response: There is really no right or wrong answer with this response because the interviewee might specialize with a certain age, gender, or style. For example, the stylist might specialize in dreadlocks.

Unsatisfactory Response: Because there is no right or wrong answer, make sure the stylist's response is in alignment with the practices of your beauty shop.

Tell me about a time you had a customer that did not like his/her haircut. What did you do to correct this issue? Did the customer return. Walk me through the process and purpose.

Satisfactory Response: Some would say the customer is always right, but that is not always the case. In this response, I would look to see if the interviewee is solution oriented or confrontational. Was the customer taken care of or if the customer return. This question would give you a picture of how the interviewee handles customers. The goal of this question is to determine how the interviewee works with customers.

Unsatisfactory Response: Anything negative that could disrupt the appearance and brand of your business is not a satisfactory answer. For example, cussing out the customer, arguing with the customer, or even showing that you have an attitude through your body language would not be satisfactory.

Where do you see yourself in 10 years?

Satisfactory Response: This answer could give you a better perspective on whether this person will be with you for the long haul or only short-term. The person you are interviewing might be an eagle and want to fly to greater heights. On the flip side, you might interview a person that just wants to do hair and not worry about owning and operating a beauty shop. Whatever the answer may be, it has to be in alignment with what you are seeking as the beauty shop owner.

Unsatisfactory Response: Not knowing where you want to be relies on the person; however, depending on how you are led, it could be an opportunity to mentor and groom that person.

What attracted you to apply to work at XYZ Beauty Shop?

Satisfactory Response: This answer could vary because people have various reasons. What is always refreshing to hear is the interviewee telling you that they researched or heard that your business is the place to be. Everyone wants to be part of a winner. In other cases, the interviewee might need a place to start. As a note, I have been around for a while and have worked for various organizations. I do not know ANYONE that is in a position of prominence that did not receive some level of assistance for someone. Whether it was from a friend, husband, wife, church or business colleague, assistance came in one form or another. I think it is important to recognize when people help you and that you continue that pattern. With that being said, I once spoke with a beauty shop owner, Lissa of All Phases Hair Salon, and she decided to open an additional location because many stylists, upon graduating, came to her for a job. She saw it as an opportunity to teach, mentor and grow them so they could be better stylists.

Unsatisfactory Response: As one who has worked in the human resource management capacity, I do not like hearing, "I just want a job." For example, I was part of a career fair in the past and I heard an applicant tell a recruit, "Give me any position" and "I don't know what I want." The recruiter kindly told him to go to the company's website and determine what he wanted. While I appreciate his honesty, he definitely needed some coaching. As the beauty shop owner, the interviewee's response is totally dependent on whether you want to groom this person or seek other candidates. It is all up to your desires.

Tell me about the professional relationships you have developed at work. How would you describe the best ones? The worst? Did they help your stylist career?

Satisfactory Response: By asking this question, you want to determine if the interviewee works well with people or not. This is a very important question because you do not want anyone that is toxic to your business.

You want people that can add value to your business and not take away from it. If the interviewee gives you clear positive answers and examples, that is a good sign. While listening to their answers, be sure to observe their facial movement and body language as those gestures can give you the positive and negative signs of what delights or annoys them.

Unsatisfactory Response: Anything negative and "I am the victim" responses are not satisfactory responses.

What's your definition of hard work and working smart? What schedule do you keep? What does your typical day look like in the salon?

Satisfactory Response: In this question you want to find out if the interviewee is organized and what that person's work ethic is. Like any profession, the time you put into a job is important, but what is more important is what you are doing while at work. Some people will brag and say I have been at work 12 hours today, but four to five of those hours included them visiting their coworkers, taking long breaks, or just flat out occupying space. You want to find out if the interviewee has a set pattern and a consistent flow of customers. If they don't, you may ask about their plan to attract new customers. You also want to determine what type of work hours they maintain. I know some people maintain various hours, but you cannot make any money working from 10 am to 2 pm. I am still a believer that the early bird gets the worm. There are customers that are willing to have a 6:00 am appointment to be styled even before work.

Unsatisfactory Response: Any response that shows lack of organization, not putting in the time, and not in alignment with the goals and objective of your business is unsatisfactory.

What is something you could do every day for the rest of your career?

Satisfactory Response: This question is to determine the interviewee's passion. I believe that when a person is passionate about something, it is not work and they can do it effortlessly.

Unsatisfactory Response: While there is no right or wrong answer, you would want to hear the interviewee give you feedback on what they love to do because it would show you that they have an X factor, something that drives them internally.

Asking questions during the interview process will eliminate many headaches as a business owner. It is like not asking questions of someone you might date. In either case, it could be a waste of time and money. We all know that some people talk a good game, so it is important to watch their ways and actions to ensure they are in alignment with your expectations. I once had a supervisor who use to say don't tell me you love me, show me. That holds true in business. Do not only tell me what you can do, show me in your work practices.

As a business owner, it is imperative that you separate personal from business. This holds true with knowing what questions you should not ask during an interview.

Asking the wrong questions are not only inappropriate, but also against the law. Below are sample questions you should not ask an interviewee.

Questions to Avoid:

- Are you married?
- What is your race and gender orientation?
- What country were you born in?
- How old are you?
- What is your religion?
- Are you disabled?

Be mindful that when you are asking questions that you are not discriminating, no matter how comfortable you become with the interviewee. If you are not comfortable with developing questions or knowing what types of questions to ask, consult a Human Resource professional. Another form of ensuring you have the right person on your team is having the stylist to go through tests to determine the skill set of styling hair. You can set up a mock situation and have the applicant cut a different style to determine the level and skill set. This might sound cumbersome, but there is nothing costlier than hiring the wrong persons and having to figure out ways to get them off your team.

While you might have great expectations of having

people on your team, you must have respect for them and have an open line of communication. While communicating, you must be transparent, honest and open to receiving feedback. One sure way to get someone on your team is to listen and value their feedback. I know this will be hard for some to do because you are the owner, but acknowledging and listening to your team members will go a long way.

As an incentive to get the right people on your team, determine what benefits you can offer team members and what it takes to attract the best team players. For instance, in addition to your chair rental, you also could offer profit sharing and business investment initiatives to build more commitment from your team members and drive business. You also could offer a 401K retirement plan and contribute a percentage based on their number of years of service. As a note, speak with a financial advisor on the different options you could offer your team members. If you are not at the position to financially support your team, you can always provide mentoring. Mentoring consists of providing professional and life guidance and instruction. This could be powerful because it strengthens trust and understanding between you and the team member.

In conclusion, it is important that you establish the right set of rules and expectations and have team members that believe in and embrace your vision. You should weigh what you can offer to incentivize your team members and determine what you can pay to invest in and strengthen your empire.

Booth Rental Agreement

Once you have selected the right team member, it is extremely important that you have a booth rental agreement. This agreement is a written legal lease contract between you and the stylist. This agreement grants permission to the stylist to use a designated area inside your business in exchange for a fee. Your agreement can be flexible according to the needs of the business. Whether you are a business owner or one renting a booth, it is important to have a written agreement in place that is signed and dated by all parties. It is important because it spells out the rules and expectations of your business. As the booth renter, it allows for you to review a document and decide if that beauty shop is right for you. The reality is you have to get into an organization to really learn its ways and customers, but if you see extreme expectations on an agreement, there is a good chance you might be walking into a burning building. Below are items that should be included in your agreement.

Description of the rental booth: This would include the space and location of the booth and if any amenities are included.

Terms of the agreement: This outlines if the agreement is weekly, monthly or yearly. It would state the start and end dates of the agreement. It would also state ramifications if the agreement in broken unexpectedly, such as a month of booth rental is not paid.

Stated responsibilities of the stylist: This outlines the beauty shop guidelines and the responsibilities the stylist.

Clauses: This outlines whether the booth renter is allowed to conduct other business within his/her booth space, such as subcontracting.

While developing a booth rental agreement is easy, be mindful that the agreement language is lawful, ethical and compliant. If you need assistance with your agreement, please consult a business professional or attorney.

Questions

- What type of stylist will be on your team?

- How do you plan to manage your team of stylists?
- What can you initially offer your stylists as a benefit?
- How often will you communicate your vision and expectations?

Chapter 5
Beauty Shop Financial Management and Business Operations

Running and operating any business requires sound financial management, and you don't need to be a finance major in order to do so. If you do not operate your business properly, the business most likely will fail. That is the reality. The beauty of running a beauty shop is that it is somewhat recession-proof. What I mean by recession-proof is this: regardless of the economy, people still need to get their hair styled and cut, because they want to look nice and be ready for the red carpet. When the economy is not good, some will look at other alternatives, but many people will continue to go to their preferred beauty shops to get styles and socialize. One beauty shop owner who has been in the business for 20 years, told me that her business has been consistent throughout those years.

Knowing the financial position of your beauty shop is not rocket science. It is a matter of knowing where your money is coming from and where it is going. I am going to go over tips, and practices and how one should look at operating the financial aspect of your business. As a business person, experience proves that it is extremely important for you to know the basics of financial management. Leaving your financial matters in the hands of others is not only unacceptable in my book but also a recipe for failure.   I am not saying you should not rely on wise counsel; I am saying your counsel should have credibility and that controls need to be put in place to safeguard your earnings. For example, every dollar and cent that is transacted should be accounted for. If you are writing checks, and you are the owner, only you should sign the checks.

What I am going to cover are some basic accounting terms and strategies so you can see the profitability of your business. I am also going to discuss paying taxes, your retirement savings, investing and protecting yourself and your business. Various software systems are available that can assist you in understanding and managing your beauty shop and your personal finances. I would advise that you purchase software such as Intuit QuickBooks or Tax Matters. In addition, seek the advice of a bookkeeper, a Certified Financial Planner (CFP), and Certified Public Accountant (CPA).

Income Statements and Cash-Flow Statements

Some basic financial statements you should look at are Income Statements and Cash-Flow statements. The income statement shows the profit and loss of your beauty shop. When you cut and style hair, the sales from cutting and styling are called income or "revenue." The supplies and equipment you purchase and utilities you pay are classified as expenses. As a business owner, chair rental will be classified as revenue because that is what you are charging stylists in your beauty shop. As a stylist working within a beauty shop, your chair rental would be classified as an expense. As a beauty shop owner, it is very important that you keep your chair or booth rentals full because that adds more revenue for the business. Using both the income statement and cash-flow statements can be a useful tool in monitoring the finances of your beauty shop.

For example, if you make $7,000 styling hair during a period of time and you spend $4,300 in expenses, your profit for that period would be $2,700. (See example.):

Example
Income Statement of XYZ Beauty Shop
for the period ending 31st December 2017

INCOME		$ 7,000.00
Services Rendered	$ 7,000.00	
EXPENSES		$ (4,300.00)
Telephone and Internet	$ 300.00	
Water and Electricity	$ 500.00	
Property Lease	$ 1,500.00	
Insurance	$ 300.00	
Advertising Cost	$ 500.00	
Taxes	$ 1,000.00	
Bank Charges	$ 200.00	
NET PROFIT		$ 2,700.00

On the other hand, if you make $7,000 styling hair during a period of time and your expenses were $8,200; your loss during that time would be $1,200.

Example
Income Statement of XYZ Beauty Shop
for the period ending 31st December 2017

INCOME		$ 7,000.00
Services Rendered	$ 7,000.00	
EXPENSES		$(8,200.00)
Telephone and Internet	$ 300.00	
Water and Electricity	$ 500.00	
Property Lease	$ 4,000.00	
Insurance	$ 500.00	
Advertising Cost	$ 500.00	
Taxes	$ 2,000.00	
Bank Charges	$ 400.00	
NET PROFIT		$(1,200.00)

As you can see, the income statement will show the different categories and how your expenses will fluctuate (variable) or remain fixed over time. For example, a mortgage or lease payment will remain the same for that period of time, unless you have an adjustable mortgage rate or you are renewing your lease. Examples of variable expenses would be your utilities and advertising costs. Now we know that if you continuously make a loss, you would be out of business soon.

Example
Cash Flow Statement of XYZ Beauty Shop
for the period ending 28th February 2017

Cash receipts from customers	$ 7,000.00
Cash paid to suppliers	$(2,000.00)
Cash generated from operations	$ 5,000.00
CASH FLOW FROM OPERATING ACTIVITIES	$ 5,000.00
CASH FLOW FROM INVESTING ACTIVITIES	
Additions to equipment	$(4,000.00)
Net cash flow from investing activities	$(4,000.00)
CASH FLOW FROM FINANCING ACTIVITIES	
Proceeds from Loan	$ 5,000.00
Payment to Loan	$ (500.00)
Net cash flow from financing activities	$ 4,500.00
NET INCREASE/DECREASE IN CASH	$ 5,500.00
Cash at the beginning of the period	$ -
Cash at the end of the period	$ 5,500.00

According to Inc., a cash-flow statement is a financial report that describes where revenue is generated at a specific period. This statement is useful in determining how functional a company is in the short-term, particularly its ability to pay bills (see earlier example). The management of your on-hand cash can be analyzed from this statement. The difference between the income statement and cash-flow statement is that the income statement considers some of the non-cash accounting items, such as depreciation. The cash-flow statement omits that and shows exactly how much actual money the business has generated. Cash-flow statements show how business has performed in managing inflows and outflows of cash. It also provides a sharper picture of a company's ability to pay creditors and finance growth.

Paying Taxes

The beauty shop business is primarily a cash business, meaning stylists accept payment in the form of cash. Many stylists have evolved to accepting payment through credit cards. When accepting payment through cash, you would have discretion in how you report your earnings. I have been told that some report their accurate amounts and others do not report it accordingly. Whether you are reporting the accurate amount or not, you do want to report it accordingly.

For starters, paying taxes is the law. There is no way to get around it. There are ways you could lower your tax liability and I advise you seek out a certified public accountant (CPA) to stay abreast of tax laws and to exercise the benefit of being a business owner. In addition, there is a way that Big Brother, that is the Internal Revenue Service (IRS), always figures out a way to catch up with you. I once facilitated a community event on entrepreneurship and one of the speakers was from the IRS. At the end of the presentation, he said, "We know who you are," meaning they know who is doing what. Now, I am not trying to scare you, and I don't believe that the IRS knows every single person that is reporting inaccurate income amounts. What I do believe is that sometimes people might cheat unknowingly or cheat intentionally, just a little, without getting caught. After not getting caught, they continue, and their cheating grows over time. As the cheating continues, it becomes more noticeable. For example, it is questionable when one reports that she makes $40,000 annually but lives in a $300,000 home and drives a 7 series BMW, when she is actually earning $90,000 annually. That situation brings attention to yourself from friends and the IRS. Sadly, there could come a time when you might get audited and have to pay back taxes, penalties, and even worse, serve time in jail.

In today's economy, receiving Social Security benefits

might not fulfill one's standard of living. There are options that one could invest in to lower their tax liability (the amount of taxes one has to pay). One such option is an Individual Retirement Account (IRA). An IRA is a type of savings account that is designed to help you save for retirement and offers many tax advantages. There are several types of IRAs: Traditional IRAs, Roth IRAs, SIMPLE IRAs and SEP IRAs. IRAs can consist of a range of financial products such as stocks, bonds or mutual funds (www.investopedia.com). A Solo 401(k), (also known as a Self Employed 401(k) or Individual 401(k)) is a 401(k) qualified retirement plan for Americans that was designed specifically for employers with no full-time employees other than the business owner(s) and their spouse(s) (money.cnn.com). There are other forms of investments that one could invest in even before retirement, such as real estate and the stock market. Investing in real estate or the stock market is an excellent way of creating wealth. If properly invested, one could speed up achieving financial goals; however, investing is a discipline and a life-time process. Whatever you decide, please seek wise counsel by speaking with a financial professional.

As you generate sales, be sure to save a portion of it. This is outside of your investments and retirement. Growing up, my parents use to tell me to always save for a rainy day and by living life, you will have those days. One strategy involves determining how much to charge your customers and adding a percentage to that amount. For example, if you charge $40 for a certain style, add 15 percent on top of that. Your new price for

Savings Strategy					
No. of customers	Price	Percentage	(Price x Percentage)	(No. of Customers x Price)	Total Savings
10	$40.00	15%	$6.00	$400.00	$60.00
20	$40.00	15%	$6.00	$800.00	$120.00
30	$40.00	15%	$6.00	$1,200.00	$180.00
40	$40.00	15%	$6.00	$1,600.00	$240.00
50	$40.00	15%	$6.00	$2,000.00	$300.00
60	$40.00	15%	$6.00	$2,400.00	$360.00
70	$40.00	15%	$6.00	$2,800.00	$420.00
80	$40.00	15%	$6.00	$3,200.00	$480.00
90	$40.00	15%	$6.00	$3,600.00	$540.00
100	$40.00	15%	$6.00	$4,000.00	$600.00

that style will be $46. That difference, $6, could go into your savings. It might not look like much, but the more customers you serve, the more money you accumulate for your savings (See savings strategy diagram).

Protecting Yourself and Business

In life we will experience great days, sick days, and all kinds of days in between. On our life journey, we are not able to predict the future. Because of the unknowns in life, it is important that we try to prepare for the unexpected. As a business owner, you have to protect yourself and your business. You have to protect yourself personally and fiscally. Insurance is one important way of protecting yourself personally. Health, disability, business and life insurances are necessary safety nets for any successful business owner.

Health Insurance

Health insurance is a must in our lives because we have to take care of ourselves. Simply put, if you don't have your health, your ability to earn a living is compromised. Health insurance covers preventive and existing conditions. With the climate of the health insurance market being debated, no one knows what direction health insurance is going in the United States. Regardless, we still have to have it. I would advise that you seek out a carrier. In addition, if you are a veteran, speak with a Veterans Administration (VA) representative to determine your level of health insurance eligibility through the VA. As a veteran, I go to the Veterans Hospital and utilize its health services.

Disability Insurance

Disability insurance covers you in case you are unable to work. Because there is only one of you and you are the source of your income, it is extremely important that you have this form of insurance (www.ssa.gov). Disability insurance offers income protection to individuals who become disabled for a long period of time, and as a result can no longer work during that time period. The premiums and benefits of disability income-protection insurance will vary, depending on your gender, age, health history, income, job and physical condition. That amount usually runs between 1 and 3 percent of your income.

Business Insurance

Business Insurance protects your business in terms of liability due to events that occur in the course of your business. There are many types of business insurance coverage; there is property damage, legal liability and employee-related risks. Why is business insurance important? It is important because it protects you from the unexpected risks of operating a business. Risks can be internal and external and come in many forms. As your business grows financially, so do your risks. At a conference I once attended, a businessman stated: the more money you make, the more people will come after your income. I believe he was telling the truth because people are drawn to money and there is that element of the population that seeks to get money by any means. Like the lyrics of P Diddy and Mase in their song, "Mo Money, Mo Problems." they were saying the more you have, the more people see you as a target for their personal gain. You have to protect yourself, your team members and your business. Speak to an insurance broker to explore the various options that are best for you.

Life Insurance

What good is starting a business when, after you pass away, the work you put into it stops? Death is one of those matter-of-fact parts of life that is going to happen, so why not consider how your work, your life and what you stand for continues? One way to ensure that your legacy continues is through life insurance. I recommend whole life insurance as it is a form of insurance that is paid out in the event of one's death. Beneficiaries are those who will be the recipients of an insurance payout. You can select anyone to be a beneficiary. I have a set of twins, a son and a daughter. When I leave this earth, I want what I stand for and believe in to continue. By providing my children insurance and other investments, I will put them in a better financial position as well as ensure that my legacy continues. What is key to ensuring that your legacy continues is teaching the recipients what you believe and stand for in life. Please seek an insurance carrier to explore your options.

Business Operations

Business operations involve how your beauty shop operates on a daily basis. The hours of operation, appointment schedule and accepted payment methods are part of your operations. I am going to discuss those three areas and explain how each could affect your revenue (sales).

Beauty Shop Hours

In any business, hours of operations are crucial because it presents an opportunity to service customers.

Whatever hours you have listed for your beauty shop, whether printed on the door, website, in ads, etc., they must be carried out. There is nothing more dejecting than for a customer to come to a business during a time open hours are listed and find the business is closed. You just lost a possible customer, and equally important, an opportunity to make money. If your business should be open and if you are unable to be there, assign one of your other stylists to open. Opening your beauty shop is important and whoever is doing it must be dependable. If your shop is advertised to open at 8 a.m., I would have the opener arrive half an hour to an hour before opening time. The opener can make sure that the building is clean on the outside and inside, the lights and equipment are working properly and any refreshments are set up and in place. Being in a service industry where customers could come in at any time, this is important. In my days of working retail management, my managers and I would do what I just discussed. We would drive around the building to make sure it was safe and clean, then prepare the building for opening. I would say to them, "No matter how we feel, when those doors open, it's show time," meaning, it is time to service customers. Whenever you open your business, you have to be consistent in its operating times. This is your business and your credibility, so be sure to follow through.

Scheduling Appointments

I have talked with countless people on how their time is valuable. As a beauty shop owner, knowing how long it takes to complete a style and scheduling your appointments directly affects the money you make. I have witnessed people in my circle of friends and family spending hours and hours at the beauty shop. They have told me that their stylist had overbooked and that is why it took so long. I have also taught beauty shop owners about time management and how to increase revenue (sales). I know making money is a priority for many, but if you want to truly maximize your money, schedule your appointments appropriately and keep them. I can imagine that overbooking your customers could be stressful to you as well, and I believe if you incorporate a scheduling system, your stress level will decrease.

Acceptance of Payment

Historically, the beauty shop business has been a cash business and customers typically pay in cash. If you are looking to expand your business, I would suggest being more versatile in the way you accept payment. Now, many salons and barber shops, are accepting credit or debit card payments. A lot of businesses use Pay Pal or Square to accept payments. This is the way of business; more importantly, it gives your customer more ways to pay you.

Questions

- Who will manage your day-to-day transactions?
- When do you plan to retire?
- Do you need a financial professional to assist you with your finances?
- What are your financial business goals?
- What are your retirement goals?
- Do you have a scheduling system in place?

Chapter 6
If I Build It, They Will Come:
Strategies for Marketing and Branding Your Beauty Shop

When you see the golden arches, what do you think of? McDonald's? When you see the red bullseye, what comes to mind? Target? There are many more images that we immediately think of because those organizations have strong brands. These strong brands would not be possible without the strategic marketing efforts that promote the organization, through various marketing channels. All businesses must market their products and services, and if you want your beauty shop business to grow, you must develop a plan to reach new and existing customers. In this section, I will discuss marketing and branding and how hey can help your beauty shop business thrive.

What Is Marketing?

Marketing is defined as the strategic activities to promote, attract and sell a product or service. Marketing operates on four spheres, called the 4Ps of marketing. The 4Ps are product, price, place and promotion.

Marketing converts strategies into sales by telling a story and getting a message across to those who want or need that product or service. That message comes in various forms — word of mouth, social media, television, billboards, newspapers, magazines, snail mail, and email — and the message is also targeted for those who need to see it.

As a beauty shop owner, how do you market your product and services and build a brand? You have to develop a strategy that includes referrals, advertising, promotions and endorsements. Even the simple tasks of sending emails or returning customer calls can be considered marketing efforts.

How Do You Market Your Beauty Shop?

Successfully marketing your beauty shop will help make your business profitable. Marketing, coupled with quality service, will convert customers into repeat customers. If your service is great, you will have customers coming from surrounding neighborhoods, because word will travel. So how do people market their beauty shops to attract customers? While there are thousands of beauty shops around, how do people make their beauty shop unique? The answer involves looking at what your competitors are doing, determining what your customers need and adding a twist to what your beauty shop offers. Oftentimes, it may seem like you have to create something new in order for people to want it. That is not the case. Adding a slight deviation to your business marketing could attract a new customer. For example, being open during nontraditional hours could attract customers who have a nontraditional work schedule. When you combine those factors, you will be on your way to applying the 4Ps to your marketing strategy.

Product

As a hair stylist, you are selling your service. In terms of marketing, you should look at your service as a product. You should view it in terms of how to present and sell it to the customer. With any product, how it is presented (its packaging) is what catches the attention of the buyer. As a business teacher, I have taught many courses discussing the importance of product presentation. I have emphasized that any product or service needs to be presented on a fine china plate and not on top of a garbage can lid. What I mean by that is you want your product or service to be appealing to the eye. To appeal to the eye as a stylist, you need to show examples of your work and your flexibility of doing different styles. You will have customers who see styles that they like from social media apps such as Pinterest and magazines. They will desire these styles, and you need to be prepared to deliver on their requests. However, if you want to set yourself apart from the rest, why not create your own personal billboard of your own creative work? You could even display additional original hairstyles. Creating your own hairstyle board would add to your presentation of work. In addition, many people promote their work through various social apps, such as Instagram and Facebook. Social media platforms provide an excellent opportunity for you to build an audience, educate them about your work and promote your products and services.

Price

Price refers to the amount that you will charge

customers for the service you provide. Your pricing strategy will play a crucial role in your marketing plan. You cannot simply grab a number out of the air and publish it. There are numerous factors to consider when pinning down your pricing strategy. It boils down to four things. The first is your cost and profit margin. You should make sure that your price will help you generate enough profit to make the business grow. The second consideration is your pricing scheme. It must be competitive, not too low and not too high. You need to research a benchmark among similar businesses in your area. Conduct a competitor price check to see how your pricing strategy will fare in the local market. Sometimes, it can make the business look cheap and, in effect, turn off potential customers. Do not be too quick to make your prices lower than your competitors. Third is your value proposition. What I mean by this is what benefit you provide for customers and how distinctly well you do it. If you have excellent customer service and offer something that your competitors do not, then a higher pricing model could be ideal. Find the middle ground, reflect on your skills and abilities, and adjust your pricing as you add or take away services. The fourth is your target customer. Defining your target customer is key. For example, if you want to charge $80 as a base price, you more than likely will be targeting the upper middle class customer. When developing prices for your services, consider the location (place); this is very important in reaching your customer and being visible.

Place

Place refers to the location of your beauty shop. As you put together your marketing plan, the location of your business will play an important role in determining the foot traffic of your beauty shop. Your beauty shop should be convenient for your target market customers. For instance, if you are targeting military personnel, then your business should be located near a military base. If your target customers are college students, then it should be near a college or university. If you are targeting corporate women, you should locate your business near corporate business hubs and have hours that accommodate their schedules.

Promotion

Promotion refers to the specific marketing steps that you

will take to tell your targeted customer about your product, price and place. You have many options. You can put out an ad in the local paper, attend trade shows or hand out flyers. You also can visit area radio stations and ask them to promote your beauty shop, or use social media sites. Make sure that you know where your target customer lives, shops, and works, and advertise in places they frequent. The above-mentioned advertisement strategies can cost a large amount of money, and sometimes you have to be creative. For instance, there is nothing like the power of marketing your business through community service and networking. The phenomenal thing about serving others and letting people know what you are doing, is that seeds are planted that position your business to attract customers. Once you attract those customers, it is up to you to water that seed so that your business will continue to grow.

During the process of determining your 4 Ps, it is important to do market research to gain information about customer needs and preferences. There is a web site (www.sizeup.com) that provides excellent insight on your industry and competitors.

What Are the Cost-Effective Ways to Market Your Beauty Shop?

All marketing efforts will cost you either money or time. You should be prepared for both if you want to let your target customer know about your beauty shop. Fortunately, promoting your business does not have to be too expensive.

One of the good things about a beauty shop is that you can build your clientele in the local market because it is very rare that a customer will drive a long way to get a haircut or style unless you are at superstar status. Usually, they only look within their local area to find a beauty shop. Therefore, your marketing reach does not have to be too far, which will cost you less.

There are various ways for you to make your marketing efforts cost-efficient. It all begins with a deeper knowledge of your target market. You need to know where your customers live, work, play and the places they frequent so you can concentrate your marketing efforts there. There is no use in promoting your business in places where nobody will be interested in going. How do you determine exactly how to promote your business in the most cost-efficient way? Here are some of your options:

- Establish partnerships with local businesses. For instance, you can give special discounts to patrons of a particular store as long as the store will allow you to put a sign to advertise there and vice versa.

- Use social media. This is one of the cheapest and most effective ways to market your beauty shop without spending too much. You simply should create a Facebook page and invite people to your site. Post activities, promotions, discounts and beauty shop events. You can post before-and-after photos of your customers so potential customers will know what your beauty shop stylists can do. Be sure to get your customers' before posting their pictures on social media.

- Find area publications and pay to include a two-for-one haircut and styling coupon inside. This could also be placed on your social media pages, enticing potential customers to visit your beauty shop to avail themselves of your services. If you price it a little higher than the usual hair style, and the second one could be free.

- Be a part of local events to promote your beauty shop, services and products. Check community listings and participate in upcoming events to promote your services. While it might be cumbersome to style someone's hair at a community event, cutting hair could be an option. I have run into countless stylists who cut hair as well style it. Having giveaways is also an excellent way of taking advantage of the exposure. For example, when it is near back-to-school time, you could give away school supplies featuring your business name and offer style and cut specials for school-age children. Feel free to hand out flyers of your price list during the event, as well as do Facebook live postings to promote and speak with customers. You might be thinking, how can I do events when I need to be in the shop styling and cutting hair? There are community and trade show models that you can hire to promote your products and services.

These are only a few of the things that you can do to market your beauty shop without spending too much. These strategies help to establish and solidify your brand.

What Is Branding?

One key ingredient in your marketing efforts is branding. Branding involves ensuring that when people see your logo, they associate it with your business. When they hear your business name, they think of your product and services, and when they think of your business, they either want to visit or avoid it. Branding allows you to instantly communicate your message to your target market. As the owner of your beauty shop, how you and team members carry yourselves is a part of your business brand. Below are questions you need to consider. Answering the questions will assist you in recognizing and establishing your brand.

- How do you see yourself and beauty shop?
- What do you offer that is unique?
- How does your business look on the outside and inside?
- What sets you apart from other beauty shops?
- How do customers view you?
- What does your customer expect from your business?

These are some of the key questions you need to address while developing your brand.

How Do You Brand Your Beauty Shop?

I have been to various beauty shops and observed many different experiences. I have been in the quiet relaxing beauty shops where customers stay to themselves and in those where a gossip hub exists. Those experiences, whether good or indifferent, have stayed with me. So, as a beauty shop owner, what experience do you want your customers to remember? It starts with branding. Let us begin with the logo. Your business logo serves as that single image that encompasses your business. Your logo should embody your business's personality and character and is the main anchor for a certain customer service mindset based on the quality of your services. If customers leave your beauty shop highly satisfied, they will equate it to your business and ultimately identify your business by its logo. This visual psychological phenomena serves as a reminder of the importance of providing great service. This also increases the chances of developing brand champions for business — customers who tell their network of family and friends about the wonderful service experience and become part of your organic marketing mix.

Another element of your brand involves curb appeal. This simply means that potential customers are enticed to physically drop in your shop because of how it looks from the outside. This can be as simple as clean windows and neon signs or even attractive exterior decor. Curb appeal helps business drive foot traffic and prompts your customers to associate your brand with a specific appeal.

Since a beauty shop is mostly geared toward women, it is a good idea to think of adjacent products that would cater to your market. Some women might want water, soda or even wine while awaiting their appointments. If your beauty shop caters to families, having a child-care service and a small space where kids can play or watch TV could be a very customer-friendly add-on. Offering free wi-fi could also create extra business. These extra services then become part of your business appeal that makes people walk through the door.

You also can incorporate convenience with your brand marketing efforts. Are you located in a fast-paced environment? If so, then you can include the availability of being able to schedule an appointment at specific times in a day. If your beauty shop is in a community where there is a population of older adults, providing a home service option could also be a great idea (check area licensing requirements first).

Regardless of how you market or brand your beauty shop, it is important to remember that you need to stay true to the identity of your business model and your target market. It will do you good to promote the business in the way that is most appealing to your target market. In summary, you will not gain customers if you fail to look appealing to your target customer, so you need to continuously find ways to determine your target market's needs and appeal to them.

Questions

- How do you plan to market your business?
- How do you plan to brand your business?
- How does your customer look (age, race, job profession, etc.)?

Chapter 7
Am I My Customer's Keeper? Customer Service and Loyalty Strategies

Your customers play an important part in the success of your business. In addition, while entry into the beauty shop industry is easy, competition is steep. Thus, you need to consider yourself as your customers' keeper. You want to make sure they are satisfied with your services because they will be the ones to bring in the money that keeps your beauty shop thriving.

In this section, I will discuss the importance of providing excellent customer service. It is extremely important to offer great customer service, even if you are having a bad day or a customer has a negative attitude. You should be mindful that you have people watching you, and overreacting could damage your reputation and business.

What Is Customer Service?

According to a recent customer engagement survey conducted by Accenture, 45 percent of customers are willing to pay more if it leads to better customer service.

In fact, the survey estimates that $1.6 trillion worth of business is lost due to poor customer service. In the beauty shop business, customer service and timing are extremely important. If you want to maintain and attract more customers, offer high quality with timely styling.

What Exactly Is This Type of Service?

Customer service is the support that you offer your customers before, during and after they receive a product or service. It refers to the effort you make to take care of customer needs. It is the protocol that you follow to provide and deliver high-quality, professional, efficient products and services.

Some businesses lose customers because they only focus on the before and during phases of the business transaction, or simply don't know how to offer quality customer service. One situation in particular that troubles me deeply is when a business owner is rude and has poor customer service but has the attitude that they are doing customers a favor by allowing them to purchase their product or service. Go figure! Even more troubling is when they fail to put any effort into providing customer support after the customer has paid for the service. And please don't even think about trying to return an item or discuss the service after the sale! If you do right by your customers, your efforts will eventually help you gain loyal ones. You will turn new customers into loyal customers. This helps you take your business to the next level.

Why Is Customer Service Important to Your Beauty Shop?

Two words that sum up the importance of customer service to your beauty shop: branding and reputation.

Branding and Reputation

Your business is service-oriented. You are selling your ability to meet the needs of your customers. You need to make sure that you provide good service and that your customers have a pleasant experience while visiting your beauty shop. This is how you can build a strong brand and reputation, not just with your target market, but also with your competitors.

So How Does Customer Service Help with Building the Brand of Your Beauty Shop?

The brand of a company is what comes to mind when customers hear of your beauty shop business. It is the expectation that your customers have toward your business. When they see the name or logo of your beauty shop, they form expectations in their minds. These expectations are often formed by the experience that they have each time they interact with your business. Every positive interaction that you have with your customer results in a favorable branding message. Of course, every interaction is defined by the quality of your customer service efforts. If you have poor customer service, that is the branding message that you will relay to your customers.

When you keep sending negative branding messages, you can bet that it will build a bad reputation for your beauty shop. In today's digital age, having a bad reputation can spread like wildfire. People will share just about anything online, especially their bad experiences. If you do not pay attention to customer service in your beauty shop, it can be the end of your business. Sometimes, all it takes is one bad experience, a well-constructed post and some shares to ruin your reputation. When that happens, you can say goodbye to new customers. It may or may not impact your number of loyal customers, but it could damage your earning potential.

As you can see, your service or prices will play an important role in attracting customers into your beauty shop. However, it is the experience that will ultimately help convert your guests into loyal customers.

What Happens If You Provide Poor Customer Service?

If you fail to pay attention to your customer service and your clients are having bad experiences in your beauty shop, several things will happen:

Negative word of mouth. You can say goodbye to one of your most effective marketing tools. Word of mouth marketing is the free advertisement that you can get from previous customers. If they have a bad experience, they will be sure to tell others. As mentioned, the digital age makes it easy for people to share their experiences. Word will quickly spread that your beauty shop fails at customer service.

Loss of new customers. The negative publicity will surely compromise your ability to get new customers. Usually, new customers will look at business reviews before trying its product or service. If your beauty shop receives negative reviews, potential customers will hesitate before they use your hair-styling services.

Damage to your existing customer base. Not only will you compromise the ability to get new customers, you also will damage your relationship with existing customers. They may continue to use your services for now, but if they experience bad customer service or if a new beauty shop opens with a better reputation, you may lose those customers as well.

Guaranteed decrease in profit. Once you start losing customers, your revenue will be affected. Obviously, your customers pay you for your services. If they stop coming, you will lose that source of revenue. Bad customer service can seriously compromise your earning potential.

Obviously, when your revenues start to decrease, it can

only go from bad to worse. The employee morale also could decrease and the stability of the business also will be compromised. If you do not act fast and improve the quality of your customer service, you might see yourself losing team members and eventually closing your beauty shop.

Fortunately, one or two bad customer-service experiences should not be the end of your business. You can still salvage it if you act quickly. People make mistakes, and sometimes that results in a bad customer experience. So, what can you do if you have an incident of bad customer service?

Start by coming up with a resolution with the affected customers. Contact them, reach out, and speak to them directly. Try not to be too defensive, especially when you know that the beauty shop and your employees are at fault. What you want to do is to clear up the situation and make attempts to satisfy the customers before they start spreading the word about their negative experience. There are times when a bad experience can land you a loyal customer but only if you know how to treat the customer and the issue correctly.

There are many ways that you can do this. You can issue a refund. You can give a coupon for a free cut or style the next time they visit. You need to give them a reason to come back so you can redeem yourself.

After resolving the issues with the customer, the next step is to investigate what went wrong. Sometimes, a bad action is all there is to it. However, there are times when the bad action is a result of a poor customer-service skill or ineffective management. Try to get to the root cause of the customer-service problem, so it will never happen again.

If bad publicity has already spread, you may want to issue an official statement to explain what happened. Now everyone may believe you, but it might convince some to give you a chance. More importantly, it shows that you are holding yourself and business accountable and have taken steps to correct it.

Different Types of Customer Services and Strategies to Create Loyalty

There are many ways to implement good customer

service in your beauty shop. To identify what will work best, you first need to know your customers. The key to making this successful is to keep in mind that you need to put the customer first. Here are a few tips that you can use for your beauty shop:

- Come up with a unique greeting. This is something that your employees will say whenever someone enters the beauty shop. You can choose to have them shout it in unison or just have the receptionist say it. This greeting should reflect the branding of your beauty shop.
- Teach your employees how to give a genuine compliment. Your beauty shop is there to make your customers look physically good. Your employees should learn how to deliver a sincere compliment because you want the customers to feel good about themselves.
- Go the extra mile with hair-care suggestions and reminders. You want the customers to feel as if you care. They do not only want to be appreciated, they also want to know that you sincerely want them to look good. Your employees should give suggestions and reminders on proper hair care.
- Offer something before the customer leaves. This can be a product or a loyalty card that offers perks and discounts. Train your employees how to offer these without sounding like a salesperson.
- Have a proper farewell spiel. What the customers hear before they leave will stick with them. Wish them a good day and encourage

> them to come back. Be sure to show them your appreciation for visiting the beauty shop.
> - Encourage your customer to pre-book his or her next appointment.

These are general ways that you can make your customers feel good while they are in your beauty shop. Remember, you want them to have the best experience while they are with you. It is your chance to prove why they need to return to your shop to avail themselves of more services.

Developing a Listing of Customers

A customer list is simply a database that contains contact information of your customers. There are several reasons why you need this list.

First, this list will allow you to connect with your customers to provide more information about your services, such as new promotions or discounts. This list also is a great way to give your customer base a nudge and earn more profit. Finally, a customer list will allow you to generate feedback and surveys that will help you improve your customer service and overall product or service offers.

Now that you know why your beauty shop needs a customer list, the next question involves ways to generate that list. Here are a couple of options:

Have a guestbook ready. Every customer that walks into your beauty shop should be encouraged to write required information in this book.

Develop a website. This website will provide potential customers with the services and products that your beauty shop offers. It should also have a "Contact Us" page where the website visitor can get in touch with your business. Make sure you give the site visitors opportunities to input their details (e.g., pop-ups, opt-in).

Create a social media page. This is proving to be one of the most effective ways to keep your target market aware of your activities. A Facebook page or a Twitter account will help you connect with your customer base. Through this portal, you can view potential customers and send them private messages to encourage them to visit your beauty shop.

Check local business listings. This is a classic way of getting a customer list. There are companies that sell consumer contact details. This will give you a cold list of customers that you can call or send a message to so they will know that your beauty shop exists.

Look at the local paper or Yellow Book. This is another classic way of generating customers. Since your target market is probably in the neighborhood, make sure to concentrate on a local listing.

Once you have a list, make sure that you start to actively connect with your customers. This will encourage them to come and visit you at the beauty shop.

Direct Mail and Email Marketing Campaigns

The best and probably most cost-efficient way to connect with your customer list is through direct mail and email marketing campaigns. According to an article published on HBR.org, an email marketing campaign will help you know within 24 hours which recipients have opened your mail. When it comes to direct mail, a study reveals that it has the higher response rate compared to an email marketing campaign, but it costs a bit more. Before you decide about using each method, let us explore each option.

Direct Mail Marketing

Direct Mail Marketing means "snail mail." You will print out your campaigns, promotions, and discounts, place them in an envelope addressed to your customer , and mail them at the post office. They will take longer to deliver, but the chances of the mail being viewed by your potential customer are higher. The downside to this process is that it ends to be more time-consuming and expensive. The key to conducting a successful direct mail marketing campaign involves timely follow-up with the mail recipient.

Email Marketing

Email marketing is the least expensive way to roll out a marketing campaign. It is also the easiest to deliver. You can draft one email and send it to hundreds or thousands of customers with just one click. It is also easiest to track. There are systems and programs that will help you identify which of the recipients have opened your email. A downside to this method lies in the fact that your is that your email will have to compete for notice with other numerous emails that the recipient gets every day. It might even end up in their spam, or junk folder. This makes the reception less likely, when compared to direct mail.

Instead of choosing between direct mail and email, it might be a good idea to use both. Without a doubt, these two methods should be a part of your marketing campaigns because they will reflect your customer-service efforts.

Questions

- How will you handle customer conflicts?
- What type of customer service strategies will you put in place?
- Who are your best customers and how do you plan to keep them?

Chapter 8
My Beauty Shop Is My Castle: Strategies on Location, Curb Appeal, and Shop Maintenance

In the 90s, I remember looking at the program "MTV Cribs" and seeing the beautiful homes and cars of stars, and their plush life would get anyone dreaming. You cannot help but be attracted to them, wanting to go inside or live in them, right? It would get anyone to dreaming.

In this section, I will discuss how the right curb appeal will help you attract customers. We will use what you have learned about marketing and branding to come up with an overall strategy to maintain and grow your beauty shop.

Why Is Location Important to Driving Business?

Location is important to businesses that sell products or provide services directly to their customers because it plays a vital role in driving customers into your business. If you are in a high traffic area, your chances for new and walk-in customers increase. Walk-in customers are vital to the success of a beauty shop. Upscale or prominent beauty shops require appointments, but if you are just starting out, you need these walk-in customers to get you through each day. This is one of the main reasons why you should choose a location that gives your beauty shop two important things: high visibility and accessibility.

High Visibility

First, the beauty shop must be highly visible. People should be able to see your business as they pass by. As much as possible, you want to choose a place that has high foot traffic, adequate parking, and is well-lit. This will help your business be visible and allow your customers to feel safe as they come to your business. Safety is always key.

Commercial businesses close to neighborhoods are a great place to start, but these are usually expensive to rent. Not only that, the competition also will be fierce. You also might find competitors in the same area.

Accessibility

The location that you choose should also be easily

accessible. Take extra care to find a place that is on a public transportation route, and easy to visit for people with disabilities. Ideally, you want your beauty shop on the lower floor. If that is not possible, make sure the stairs or elevator can easily be used and will not hinder customers from reaching your business.

These two suggestions will help you get as many walk-in customers as possible. You also should be sure that your business location is convenient for your target market customers. For instance, if you want to cater to families, setting up your beauty shop in a mall would be a great idea. If your target market is students, you want to stay near college campuses or universities. The location of your beauty shop also will play a role in defining your desired business image and brand.

Cleanliness Is a Virtue: Benefits of a Clean Beauty Shop

Once you have selected the right location for your beauty shop, you also should consider how you will set up the business. We won't discuss the beauty shop layout just yet. We want to start with the cleanliness of your beauty shop.

Let's face it. A beauty shop can get very dirty quite fast. You style and cut hair after all. It gets everywhere. Not only that, the other services that you offer will make a mess as well. You want to make sure that you can keep your beauty shop clean and sanitized. The way you present your beauty shop speaks volumes about the service that you offer. If you cannot even maintain cleanliness in your shop, then how can the customers trust you to make their hair look good?   It really pays to have someone in your shop to make sure that the shop is consistently clean, including cleaning the floors and rest rooms. Most important, from a health and safety perspective, you want to make sure all areas of your beauty shop are sanitized.

Of course, sanitation of the tools is mandatory. Are your scissors, blades, flat irons, and other tools clean? No customer would want to have your tools touch them if the tools are not cleaned and properly sanitized. You do not have to make a show of cleaning your tools in front of your customers, but make sure they look presentable. Make sure that the cleanliness in your beauty shop adheres to health and safety standards.

Apart from the overall cleanliness and sanitation, make sure your beauty shop is also organized and in order. A well-kept shop speaks volumes about the owner and those working there. The way your tools and hair products are arranged can help boost the overall shop ambiance.

Strategies for Maintaining an Attractive Place for the Customer

When decorating your beauty shop, there are two things that you need to consider: your customers and your services. Since your customers are mostly women, you need to think about what is appealing and attractive to them. You should choose the right colors that will make them want to come back to your shop. For instance, bright colors and feminine shades like pink and lavender may be more appropriate compared to grays, blue, and earth colors.

Thinking about your customers will help you choose the right equipment and appliances. For instance, a soft high-back chair is a great choice since your customers can relax their backs while getting a style or haircut. If you cater to children, you should have one chair that is small enough for them or a highchair for them.

Some beauty shops are really upscale. While you might not decide to have chandeliers, your shop décor should be appealing and allow you to perform services efficiently. You want enough space to move around and support a natural flow for additional services that may be available. As your beauty shop grows and expands, you will probably add more services. Make sure there is room for shop upgrades.

One area that you need to pay special attention to is the waiting area. When you start getting more customers or if they come all at once, make sure that they are comfortable while they wait. Otherwise, they might get up and leave to avail themselves of the services of another shop. Choose comfortable chairs and provide entertainment or reading material to keep them occupied while waiting for their appointments.

Questions

- List areas that need to be cleaned. How often is this done?
- Whose responsibility is it to keep the beauty shop clean?

- List the supplies you need to keep the beauty shop clean. Who will order them?

Chapter 9
Using Technology to Operate Your Business and to Reach and Grow Your Customer Base

Technology is aggressively taking over every phase of our society. If you fail to integrate technology into your business, it might compromise your ability to compete in the market. Not only that, it might be more difficult to maintain and retain your customers.

In this section, I will explore the different ways that you can use technology to make your day-to-day business processes easier and more efficient.

CRM Software

CRM, or Customer Relationship Management, is a term used to refer to the strategies, programs and practices that your beauty shop should implement to help you analyze and manage all your customer data and interactions.

Any form of technology that you will use in your business will be for the benefit of your customers. If it makes your business operations easier to manage, it will help you improve your customer focus. When your customers are happy, you can expect them to return and be loyal to you. But the question is, what is the role of CRM in making your customers happy?

CRM systems are designed to help you manage your customer data so you can study and analyze what they want out of your business. It will allow you to identify the services that they prefer and those they don't. Once you know the services they are interested in, you can focus on improving them, so your customers will have a better experience in your beauty shop as they avail themselves of the products and services that you offer. Here are examples of how your CRM can help in your beauty shop:

- Organize customer information and contact details.
- Manage appointments to avoid double-booking.
- Set up reminders for upcoming appointments both for your beauty shop and the customer.
- Deliver news about new beauty shop products, services, promos and discounts.
- Update customers about schedules and holidays that can affect business operations.

These are only some of the ways that CRM can help. It is important that you to choose the system that best suits your beauty shop business processes.

Email Campaigns

Emails are a great marketing tool for your beauty shop because they allow you to implement continuous marketing campaigns.

Of course, email campaigns are more than the newsletter or content that you send out to your customer mailing list. You must know what type of emails you will send so they can be translated into customer transactions. So how do create an email campaign? Here are the steps that you need to follow:

- Get the email address of your customers. New customers should be asked to input their data, specifically their name and contact details.
- Send a personalized email to every current customer. This email is a great way to make customers feel as if they are welcomed back into the beauty shop and that you remember the services they received.
- Send an email of appreciation Send automated reminders to the customer. Men usually need to have their hair cut more often than women. You may want to send bi-weekly reminders for the next haircut, etc.
- Deliver your message of thanks and feel free to include details about services or products that the customers can use the next time they visit. To make it personalized, you may want to include hair-care tips for the customer.

- Choose coupons or discounts and send them to the customer to encourage them to visit your beauty shop once more.

Feel free to keep doing this. Sending emails to your customers will remind them that you are always available to provide your services when they need you the most; just don't bombard or overwhelm them.

Customer Rewards Program

A rewards program is a great way to encourage loyalty and continuous patronage from your customers. You will reward them for always choosing your beauty shop for their hair-care requirements.

Here are some tips to consider:

- Create different reward levels based upon number of customer visits.
- Give customers an incentive to return. For instance, if they visit your shop within the next two weeks, they get a discount or a free product or service (e.g., free massage).
- Encourage them to bring a friend. A referral reward can come in the form of a discount or a free service.
- Come up with a stamp card that will reward continuous patronage. For instance, after 10 visits, they get the 11th for free. This stamp card also can be in the form of a mobile app for easier tracking.

When creating a loyalty program for your beauty shop, it is very important to keep your customers in mind. After all, you want to create a program that will appeal to them.

Questions

- Do you have a system in place to monitor and track your customers?
- What is your goal for attracting and retaining customers?
- What customer rewards programs can you put in place to increase customer loyalty?

Chapter 10
What's Next?
Using Innovation to Grow Your Beauty Shop

Constant evaluation and evolution are the keys to keeping your beauty shop ahead of the competition. You must learn how to innovate. You need to look for ways to improve your beauty shop, evaluate your services, and take it to the next level. They may come in the form of a service or product upgrade, a renovation or a training program. These will help improve something in the business so you can increase productivity and profitability.

In this section, I will discuss the importance of training your employees and how to expand your beauty shop.

Investing in Training Staff and Expanding Expanding Locations

The growth of your beauty shop can be manifested in two ways: your staff and your beauty shop locations. Each of these will require you to invest some money and time. Let us discuss why it is worth the investment.

Training Staff

In order to offer the best service possible, you need to make sure that your staff is well-trained and able to attend to the   needs of your customers. Make sure your staff knows your expectations for how customers should be treated at all times, including your expectations for how customer complaints and negative feedback are handled. While you may be lucky to have a team full of naturally charming people, you can be sure that even they will experience a dissatisfied customer from time to time. There are stylists who may be talented in styling and cutting hair, but unable to handle a demanding, difficult customer. Train them on how to handle different kinds of customers while offering solutions to keep a customer's business. A number of options could help preserve the relationship and maintain the client's business. The stylist could introduce the client to another team member who may be a "better fit," the option of scheduling the client at a time when there can be more one-on-one interaction or scheduling a private consultation to better meet the client's needs.

In addition to providing customer service instruction for

your team, you also should invest in haircut and style skills training. Even men have evolving hairstyles and you want to make sure that your stylists can meet customer demands.

Whenever you have new programs or systems that need to be implemented, invest in training your staff for these upgrades. This is how they will learn to properly use the programs and systems. The change might take some time to get used to, so you want to give your staff enough training to make this possible.

Expanding Locations

Another sign of a growing business is expansion. In your beauty shop, it could mean renovating your current location or opening a new one in another community. Sometimes, renovating the current beauty shop is enough to give your present customer base something new to experience. Opening another additional beauty shop in another location could be profitable; however, I would first ensure that your main location is profitable. Of course, this is easier said than done. There is much to consider when investing in a new location. It is very costly and you would practically start from scratch.

You'd need to process a new set of documents, market your beauty shop in the new community, and gain the trust of the people in that area. You will be risking much, so you need to ensure that your beauty shop will be appealing enough for the new market and potential clients that you will target.

The Cost and Benefits in Expanding Your Business

The expense of your beauty shop expansion will depend on what you need to do. Try not to assume that you will be spending the same amount of money as when you opened your first beauty shop. You can only use it as a benchmark.

First, construction costs may have increased since your last opening. Obviously, you need to hire a contractor to build or renovate your new beauty shop. The labor cost might be higher compared to the time when you established your first shop. You might decide to lease; rental prices could be higher. Owning or leasing is a decision you would have to make.

You also should consider the new location. Are the costs higher or lower in that neighborhood? Can you establish the same price points as your first shop? That would really depend on what your customers can afford and what the competition in that area offers.

While this investment will put a dent in your finances, there are many benefits to expanding your operations in another location. You will be tapping into a new market, and that means possibly more customers. If you can build an army of loyal customers, you can quickly double your profits. Although the overhead will increase, the potential to earn also will go up.

Another benefit that you can expect is publicity. The opening of a beauty shop creates a "buzz" that also can benefit your other establishment. As you advertise your new location, you are bound to mention your other shop and that can give your profits a boost. Of course, you should make sure that your calculations will be done smartly and carefully. Although you will be spending, make sure that it will be less than your expected earnings. You need to work on the return of this new investment if you want to continue growing your beauty shop.

Questions

- How often do you evaluate your beauty shop and its position of growth and expansion?
- Where is the ideal location to place and expand your beauty shop?
- If you plan to expand, when?

Conclusion

I believe that beauty shops are going to be around   until the end of time. While the fundamentals and craft of styling remain basically unchanged, how one attracts a customer is key. Today's customer is often on the go, so offering more timely services would is more attractive to customers. We see this strategy in corporations that own beauty shops as they offer various services to meet customer needs. I call this level of service a one-stop-shop business, and I see this expanding in the future. To be a one-stop-shop beauty shop, you must offer what your customers need. However, you must know your customers' habits, likes and dislikes. For example, you cannot offer high-end products to a moderately income-based clientele. In essence, there are three sure-fire ways to make certain that your beauty shop continues to thrive. One, whatever you offer should be in alignment with and attractive to your target market. Two, you must be able to take a risk by introducing something new. Three, make sure whatever you offer is visually appealing. You want to offer your products and services on a china plate instead of a garbage can lid. Presentation is key in all types of sales.

As you work and grow your business, it is my hope that

you utilize the material in this book. The beauty shop business is a great profession, and there is an enormous opportunity to make a great deal of money. The success and direction of your beauty shop is up to you. You are the owner and driver of this luxury vehicle! While I do not expect you to use every tip in this book, the action steps below are paramount to the success of your business:

- Develop and execute a plan for your beauty shop. Always plan everything you do.
- Seek guidance regarding things you don't understand.
- Do not spend every penny you make. Save for emergencies, retirement, savings and paying yourself.
- Always network, build business relationships and serve your community.
- Always do the right thing, and I dare you to do it right!

All the best in your future endeavors!

About the Author

As a lifelong visionary and community advocate, Alan D. Benson is the founder and president of Benson Group, LLC, a human resources company that specializes in workforce training, professional recruitment and project management services. He has more than 25 years of experience in operations management, training and development and education. He has managed and empowered teams, created and facilitated trainings, and developed systems to streamline operations for major corporations throughout the U.S.

Alan is experienced and passionate about helping others reach their true potential, living a purposeful life and learning. He believes that every experience and job we have had in life helps to shape our identity, attitude and journey in life and that it is up to us to recognize the reasoning for those experiences, learn from them, and apply them to our purpose in life. This belief is his driving force in Benson Group, LLC's goal to equip individuals and companies to reach their true potential and business goals.

Alan earned a Bachelor of Science degree in Political Science and Master of Public Administration (MPA) degree from the University of Louisville. He later earned a Master of Business Administration (MBA) degree from Indiana University. He served in the U.S. Marine Corps and is a Persian Gulf War veteran. He has twins, Hilton and Hayley, and resides in Louisville, KY.

References

http://smallbusiness.chron.com/make-booth-rent-agreement-14450.html
(www.ibisworld.com, page 19). IBISWorld Industry Report OD4410
Hair Salons in the US, Competitive Landscape, page 19).
 (http://www.history.com/topics/black-history/madame-c-j-walker, 1991).
https://www.ssa.gov/disability/
http://money.cnn.com/retirement/guide/selfemployment_individual401k.moneymag/index.htm
https://www.investopedia.com/terms/i/ira.asp?adtest=rira-layout-bttn-bsln
https://www.medicare.gov/sign-up-change-plans/decide-how-to-get-medicare/whats-medicare/what-is-medicare.html
https://www.entrepreneur.com/article/223126
http://www.investopedia.com/terms/m/marketing.asp
http://www.purelybranded.com/insights/the-four-ps-of-marketing/
http://smallbusiness.chron.com/market-Beautyshop-10568.html
https://www.sba.gov/blogs/sole-proprietorship-popular-business- structure-right-you
https://www.desk.com/success-center/customer-service
https://www.accenture.com/us-en/insight-digital-disconnect- customer-engagement
http://www.investopedia.com/terms/c/customer-service.asp
https://www.retailcustomerexperience.com/blogs/why-customer- service-and-branding-are-the-same-thing/
https://www.ballantine.com/3-reasons-why-a-customer-mailing- list-is-important/
http://smallbusiness.chron.com/build-customer-list-21992.html
http://www.bluefountainmedia.com/blog/direct-mail-

marketing- and-email-marketing/
https://www.standishsalongoods.com/masculine-
Beautyshop-decor
http://www.ehow.com/how_10064334_decorate-
Beautyshop.html
https://www.biznessapps.com/blog/why-every-hair-
salon-and-
Beauty shop-needs-a-business-app/
http://searchcrm.techtarget.com/definition/CRM
http://blog.marketo.com/2014/05/instagram-
Beautyshops- and-the-power-of-continuous-
marketing.html
http://www.startabarbers.co.uk/expanding-barber-
shop- business.html
http://www.capitolhillseattle.com/2015/03/rudys-
Beautyshop- opening-on-15th-ave-e/comment-page-1/